POLYCYSTIC OVARIAN SYNDROME (PCOS) MANAGEMENT DIET COOKBOOK

Nourishing Recipes For Balanced Hormones: Delicious Meals For Optimal Health Empowering -Your Wellness Journey

DR. SHAYLA LEWIS

Table of Contents

DISCLAIMER

Write a brief complete Disclaimer for my diet cook book telling them that the author is not in any association with any company, business or individual and also this book is written by the authors knowledge and understanding

The information provided in this diet cookbook is based on the author's personal knowledge and understanding. The author is not affiliated with, endorsed by, or associated with any company, business, or individual. The recipes and dietary advice contained within this book are intended for informational purposes only. Readers should consult with a healthcare professional or a registered dietitian before making any significant changes to their diet or lifestyle. The author assumes no responsibility for any adverse effects that may result from the use or misuse of the information contained in this book.

CHAPTER ONE

Understanding PCOS: A Brief Overview

PCOS is a hormonal condition affecting the ovaries. It is distinguished by irregular periods, elevated levels of androgens (male hormones), and polycystic ovaries. Despite the name, not all people with PCOS have cysts on their ovaries.

What is PCOS?

PCOS is a complex disorder with several underlying causes. While the specific reason is unknown, genetics, insulin resistance, and hormone imbalance play important roles. Women with PCOS frequently have elevated insulin levels, which can contribute to increased androgen synthesis by the ovaries. This imbalance in hormone levels disrupts the menstrual cycle and might cause reproductive issues.

PCOS symptoms vary from person to person, ranging from minor to severe. Common symptoms include irregular menstrual periods, excessive hair growth (hirsutism), acne, weight gain, and trouble reducing weight. Some people notice hair loss on their scalps as well as skin discoloration, particularly in skin folds.

Impact on Daily Life

PCOS can significantly affect daily living, both physically and mentally. Inconsistent menstrual periods and hormonal swings can cause physical discomfort, while related symptoms like acne and hirsutism can lower self-esteem and confidence. Furthermore, reproductive concerns and long-term health complications such as diabetes and heart disease can cause severe worry and anxiety.

Diet is important for managing PCOS.

Diet is important for controlling PCOS symptoms and promoting overall health. Because insulin resistance is a typical aspect of PCOS, following a diet that regulates blood sugar levels can be useful. A diet rich in whole, unprocessed foods, high in fiber, and well-balanced in macronutrients (carbohydrates, protein, and fat) can help regulate blood sugar and increase insulin sensitivity.

Dietary recommendations for PCOS management.

Concentrate on Complex Carbohydrates: Select whole grains, fruits, vegetables, and legumes over refined carbohydrates such as white bread and sugary snacks. Complex carbs provide long-lasting energy and assist in keeping blood sugar levels stable.

Prioritise Protein: Incorporate lean protein sources into your meals, such as poultry, fish, tofu, and legumes. Protein keeps you feeling full and satisfied, which might help with weight management.

Healthy Fats: Include avocados, nuts, seeds, and olive oil in your diet. Healthy fats are necessary for hormone synthesis and can help lower inflammation.

Limit your intake of sugary meals and beverages, as these can produce abrupt rises in blood sugar levels and contribute to insulin resistance.

Manage Portion Sizes: Be conscious of portion sizes to avoid overeating and encourage weight management. Meals that are balanced in terms of carbohydrates, protein, and fat can help regulate appetite and keep blood sugar stable.

Stay Hydrated: Drink plenty of water throughout the day to maintain hydration and overall health.

Setting Realistic Goals.

Setting realistic goals is critical to successfully managing PCOS through dietary and lifestyle modifications. It's critical to approach goal-setting with patience, acknowledging that progress may be slow and setbacks are common. Here are some tips for developing realistic goals:

Start Small: Make small, attainable improvements to your food and lifestyle. Focus on one or two improvements at a time to avoid overwhelm and boost your chances of success.

Be Specific: Set clear, quantifiable, and attainable goals. Instead of saying "I want to eat healthier," you may add "include at least one serving of vegetables with every meal."

Monitor Your Progress: Keep track of your dietary choices, physical activity, and any changes in symptoms. This can help you recognize patterns, keep accountable, and celebrate your accomplishments along the road.

Seek Support: Don't be reluctant to ask for help from healthcare experts, friends, or support groups. A helpful network may offer encouragement, motivation, and direction as you strive towards your goals.

Be Flexible: Be willing to adapt your goals as needed based on your progress and circumstances. It is acceptable to adjust and modify your strategy over time to better meet your needs and preferences.

Individuals can take proactive actions to improve their health and quality of life by understanding PCOS, recognizing the role of diet in its management, and setting reasonable goals.

How Diet Influences PCOS Symptoms

Our eating choices can have a direct impact on the symptoms of PCOS. Insulin resistance is a typical characteristic of PCOS, causing high blood sugar levels and increased insulin production. High insulin levels cause the ovaries to create more androgens, worsening symptoms such as acne, excessive hair growth, and irregular menstrual cycles. As a result, concentrating on a diet that regulates blood sugar levels and insulin sensitivity is critical in managing PCOS.

CHAPTER TWO

Importance of Balanced Nutrition.

To preserve general health and effectively manage symptoms, women with PCOS must eat a well-balanced diet. Whole, nutrient-dense foods like fruits, vegetables, lean meats, and healthy fats can give the body the vitamins, minerals, and antioxidants it needs for optimal performance. Balancing macronutrients, such as carbohydrates, proteins, and fats, can help regulate blood sugar levels and minimize insulin surges.

Exploring low-carb, antioxidant-rich, and anti-inflammatory meals

Low-carbohydrate diets have shown potential in improving insulin sensitivity and lowering androgen levels in women with PCOS. Individuals with PCOS can improve their blood sugar control and lower insulin resistance by limiting their consumption of refined carbohydrates and sweets such as white bread, spaghetti, and sugary snacks.

Antioxidant-rich foods like berries, leafy greens, and nuts can help counteract the oxidative stress and inflammation associated with PCOS. Including these foods in your diet can help to balance your hormones and lower your risk of PCOS problems including cardiovascular disease and infertility.

Similarly, eating anti-inflammatory foods like fatty fish, curcumin, and olive oil can help ease PCOS symptoms by lowering inflammation in the body. Chronic inflammation is known to lead to insulin resistance and hormone abnormalities, hence anti-inflammatory foods are an important part of a PCOS management regimen.

Nourishing your body with nutrient-dense foods is critical for supporting healing and restoring balance in PCOS. Instead of perceiving food as just subsistence, think of it as medication for your body. Each meal is an opportunity to nourish your body and combat PCOS symptoms.

Consuming a variety of colorful fruits and vegetables guarantees that you get a diverse range of vitamins, minerals, and antioxidants that are necessary for hormone balance and overall wellness. Lean proteins including poultry, fish, tofu, and beans include amino acids required for hormone production and tissue repair.

Avocados, nuts, seeds, and olive oil include healthy fats that enhance hormone synthesis and induce satiety, thus regulating appetite and preventing overeating. Prioritizing nutrient-dense meals and mindful eating practices can nourish your body from the inside while also supporting its natural healing processes.

Finding Joy in Cooking and Eating Well. While controlling PCOS through nutrition may appear difficult at first, it can also serve as an opportunity to experiment with new foods, flavors, and culinary styles. Finding delight in cooking and eating can change your perspective on food and improve your overall health.

Experimenting with recipes that emphasize whole, unprocessed ingredients allows you to find delicious and enjoyable meals that help you achieve your health objectives. Experiment with different herbs, spices, and cooking methods to add flavor to your dishes without using too much salt or sugar.

Involving friends and family in dinner preparation can also make cooking an enjoyable and social activity.

Consider having a cooking night where you can share ideas, and suggestions, and eat healthy meals together.

By cultivating a positive relationship with food and enjoying the pleasure of eating healthily, you may empower yourself to take charge of your health and thrive despite PCOS.

Getting Started: Essential Kitchen Tools and Ingredients

Beginning a quest to address Polycystic Ovarian Syndrome (PCOS) through food necessitates a strategic approach to kitchen stocking. Here's how you get started with key kitchen gear and ingredients:

Essential Kitchen Tools:

A high-quality blender is ideal for creating nutritious smoothies with PCOS-friendly ingredients such as leafy greens, berries, and protein-rich Greek yogurt.

Use a non-stick skillet or grill pan to cook lean foods like chicken breast, fish, and tofu without adding oil or fat.

Use a steamer basket to cook veggies while keeping nutrition and color.

Food scales and measuring cups are essential for proper portion control and controlling PCOS-related insulin resistance.

Invest in high-quality knives and cutting boards for effortless chopping of fresh produce during dinner prep.

Key Ingredients for A PCOS-Friendly Pantry: Choose complex carbs like quinoa, brown rice, oats, and whole wheat pasta to regulate blood sugar levels and increase fullness.

Increase omega-3 fatty acid intake with foods like salmon, walnuts, flaxseeds, and avocado to lower inflammation linked to PCOS.

Choose lean proteins such as fowl, fish, tofu, tempeh, and lentils to promote muscle health and moderate hunger.

Fill your cupboard and fridge with colorful fruits and vegetables high in vitamins, minerals, and antioxidants to reduce PCOS symptoms and improve overall health.

Choose low-glycemic index (GI) foods, such as sweet potatoes, lentils, chickpeas, and berries, to regulate insulin levels and minimize blood sugar increases.

Must-Have Kitchen Gadgets for Easy Cooking

Efficient meal preparation is essential for keeping a PCOS-friendly diet. Here are some must-have kitchen devices that will help you cook more efficiently:

An Instant Pot reduces cooking time for cereals, beans, and stews while maintaining nutrients and flavors, making it ideal for busy folks.

Its adaptability enables one-pot meals with lean proteins, nutritious grains, and veggies, making it great for batch cooking and meal planning.

Air fryer:

With an air fryer, you can enjoy crispy, tasty dishes without using too much oil or fat.

Prepare healthier alternatives to traditional fried dishes, such as chicken tenders, sweet potato fries, and veggie chips, to reduce calories and fat while fulfilling appetites.

Spiralizer:

Spiralize veggies like zucchini, carrots, and sweet potatoes to create nutritious noodles.

Increase the diversity and originality of PCOS-friendly meals by creating low-carb and gluten-free pasta alternatives.

A food processor is a versatile tool for creating nutritious and delectable meals, including homemade nut butter, energy balls, creamy sauces, and dips.

Use the chopping, blending, and pureeing capabilities to easily incorporate whole foods into your PCOS control diet.

By investing in these kitchen devices, you may make meal preparation easier, diversify your menu, and keep on track with your PCOS control goals.

Incorporating Fresh Produce and Lean Protein

Putting fresh produce and lean proteins first in your meals is an important part of treating

PCOS through nutrition. Here's how to include these critical nutrients in your everyday diet:

Fresh produce:

Fill half of your plate with colorful fruits and vegetables at each meal to increase nutritional intake and satiety.

Use seasonal produce to create unique and savory dishes, such as roasted root vegetables in the fall and crisp salads with summer fruit.

Incorporate fruits and vegetables into major dishes, snacks, and desserts for a balanced diet.

Lean proteins:

Choose lean protein sources including skinless poultry, fish, tofu, tempeh, and lentils to promote muscle health and manage blood sugar levels.

Add diversity to your meals by experimenting with cooking methods such as grilling, baking, and stir-frying that are both light and nutritious.

Plant-based proteins such as quinoa, lentils, chickpeas, and edamame offer important nutrients and fiber without the saturated fat found in animal products.

You may support your PCOS control goals while also enjoying delicious and satisfying meals if you eat plenty of fresh produce and lean proteins.

Understanding Label Reading for Healthier Options

Navigating the grocery store aisles can be daunting, especially when attempting to make healthier choices to control PCOS. Here's how to interpret food labels and make the best decisions for your health:

Select goods with brief ingredient lists and recognizable whole-food ingredients.

Beware of hidden sugars, artificial additives, and preservatives that may worsen insulin resistance and inflammation in PCOS.

Consider the amount of sugar, fiber, and protein per serving to make informed choices about carbohydrate quality and portion size.

Stabilize blood sugar levels and induce fullness by choosing food strong in fiber and protein.

Be cautious of items labeled "low-fat" or "fat-free," as they may contain sugars and fillers to compensate for flavor.

For hormone balance and satiety, consume whole-fat dairy products and healthy fats such as avocado, almonds, and olive oil.

CHAPTER THREE

Choose foods with a low glycemic index (GI) to stabilize blood sugar levels by slowing carbohydrate digestion and absorption.

Eat whole grains, legumes, fruits, and vegetables with low GI to regulate insulin resistance and alleviate PCOS symptoms.

By being a skilled label reader, you may make better grocery store decisions and support your PCOS control goals with nutrient-dense, complete foods.

Meal Planning Tips for Success

Meal planning is an effective technique for sticking to your PCOS treatment diet and avoiding the temptation of harmful convenience meals. Here are some suggestions for effective meal planning:

Set aside one day per week to plan meals, make a shopping list, and prepare items ahead of time.

Use meal planning apps or templates to create a well-balanced weekly menu.

Prepare essentials like grains, meats, and roasted vegetables on weekends for convenient weekday dinners.

Prepare snacks and ingredients for smoothies or salads ahead of time for easy access to healthy options.

Select recipes with similar ingredients to reduce waste and save time and money at the grocery shop.

Use leftover components to create new dishes, such as soups, stir-fries, or salads.

Stay flexible and be kind to yourself.

Be flexible and adapt your food plan as needed to accommodate life's unexpected changes.

Develop self-compassion, prioritize progress over perfection, and celebrate accomplishments along the way.

By adopting these meal planning techniques into your daily routine, you may simplify your PCOS management diet, save time and money, and position yourself for success in meeting your health objectives.

Overcoming Common Challenges and Roadblocks

Managing PCOS can be difficult, especially when dealing with common issues including hormone fluctuations, mood swings, and unpredictable symptoms. In this chapter, we'll investigate solutions to address these obstacles, including:

Understanding hormonal imbalances: PCOS is defined by high levels of androgens (male hormones) and insulin resistance. Understanding how hormone imbalances affect your body allows you to modify your diet and lifestyle choices to control your symptoms.

Establishing a support network: Dealing with PCOS can be difficult at times, but you don't have to do it alone. Creating a support network of friends, family, and healthcare experts can offer you the encouragement and guidance you need to keep going on your path.

Setting realistic goals is critical for long-term success in treating PCOS. Instead of looking for big changes overnight, make small, long-term modifications to your food and lifestyle.

Practicing self-care is critical for treating PCOS, both physically and mentally. Resting, relaxing, and engaging in enjoyable activities can help relieve stress and increase general well-being.

Addressing Cravings and Emotional Eating
Many people who have PCOS struggle with cravings and emotional eating. Hormonal imbalances frequently cause desires for sugary and high-carbohydrate foods, but mental stress can lead to binge eating episodes. In this chapter, we'll look at techniques to deal with cravings and emotional eating, including:

Identifying triggers: Recognising the factors that cause cravings and emotional eating is the first step in overcoming these behaviors. Keep a food journal to monitor your eating habits and find patterns that may be causing your cravings.

Finding healthy alternatives: Rather than succumbing to unhealthy cravings, stock your kitchen with nutritious alternatives that will fulfill your cravings without jeopardizing your diet. For example, choose fresh fruit over sugary snacks, or air-popped popcorn over chips.

Mindful eating is the practice of paying attention to your body's hunger and fullness cues while eating with intention and awareness. Slowing down and savoring each bite helps you avoid overeating and make healthier meal choices.

Managing stress: Stress is a significant cause for emotional eating, therefore learning appropriate stress management techniques is critical for PCOS management. Deep breathing, meditation, and yoga are all relaxation techniques that can help you reduce stress and improve your emotional health.

Balancing the obligations of work, family, and personal life can be difficult, especially while attempting to manage PCOS properly. In this chapter, we'll discuss techniques to assist you in handling time constraints and busy schedules while prioritizing your health, such as:

Meal planning and preparation: Planning and preparing meals ahead of time will help you save time and guarantee that you have nutritious options on hand when you're short on time. Set up one day per week to meal prep, and batch prepare big quantities of meals that can be quickly reheated throughout the week.

Quick and easy dishes: Look for recipes that take little time and effort to make. Choose simple, nutritious meals that can be prepared in under 30 minutes, such as stir-fries, salads, and sheet pan dinners.

Utilising convenience foods: While whole, unprocessed meals are preferable, there are numerous healthy convenience foods available to help you save time in the kitchen. Fill your cupboard with canned beans, frozen vegetables, pre-cooked grains, and nutritious convenience meals that you can quickly incorporate into your meal plan.

Setting limits entails learning to say no to activities and obligations that deplete your time and energy while prioritizing activities that promote your health and wellbeing. Delegate responsibilities wherever possible, and don't be hesitant to ask for assistance when you need it.

Eating healthy on a budget is doable with proper preparation and buying tactics. In this chapter, we will cover techniques for budget-friendly shopping and meal planning, including:

Planning your meals: Before going to the grocery store, spend some time planning your week's meals. Make a list of the ingredients you'll need for each meal, and stick to it to prevent buying impulsive items.

Shopping in season: Purchasing fruits and vegetables in season not only saves money but also assures that you are obtaining the freshest food available. To save money on produce, go to your local farmers' market or seek for bargains and discounts at the grocery store.

Buying in bulk: Purchasing pantry staples like grains, beans, and nuts in bulk is generally less expensive than buying them in smaller quantities. Look for bulk bins at your grocery store, or try joining a wholesale club to save money on everyday necessities.

Cooking in batches: Batch cooking is an excellent method for saving time and money in the kitchen. Prepare large batches of meals and divide them into individual servings that may be frozen and reheated as required. This not only saves money on materials but also helps to prevent food waste.

Handling Social Situations and Dining Out
Navigating social situations and dining out can be difficult when attempting to control PCOS, but with the correct tactics, you can stay on track while still spending time with friends and family. In this chapter, we'll

discuss tips for dealing with social situations and eating out, including:

Planning ahead: Before attending social events or dining out, investigate the menu to find healthy selections that match your dietary habits and goals. If feasible, recommend eateries that have a variety of options to meet diverse dietary requirements.

Making substitutes: Do not be hesitant to request substitutions or changes to menu items to make them more PCOS-friendly. Request grilled vegetables instead of fries, or ask for dressing on the side to keep portion sizes under control.

Portion management: Portion sizes in restaurants are frequently significantly bigger than what you would eat at home, therefore it is critical to exercise portion control when dining out. Consider splitting an entree with a buddy or taking half of your meal home as leftovers.

Bringing your own food: If you're going to a potluck or dinner party, consider bringing a PCOS-friendly dish to share with others. This guarantees that you have at least one healthy option to choose from and helps others understand your dietary preferences and constraints.

Maintaining motivation on your PCOS journey can be difficult, especially when dealing with setbacks or slow progress. In this chapter, we'll look at techniques to help you stay motivated and dedicated to your health goals, including:

Celebrating minor successes: Rather than focusing entirely on the end objective, acknowledge the small victories along the route. Every accomplishment is worth celebrating, whether it's shedding a few pounds, sticking to your eating plan for a week, or noticing an increase in your energy levels.

Finding inspiration: Surround yourself with sources of inspiration that remind you of why you're determined to manage PCOS. This could include encouraging phrases, success stories from others who have overcome similar obstacles, or visual reminders of your health objectives.

Tracking your progress: Record your food, activity, and symptoms in a journal or app. Seeing how far you've come can help you stay motivated and focused on your goals, even during difficult times.

Seeking help: Don't be afraid to ask for help when you need it. Whether it's talking to a friend, attending a support group, or engaging with a healthcare professional, having a support system in place can offer you the encouragement and guidance you need to keep going on your PCOS journey.

By addressing these major issues in the Polycystic Ovarian Syndrome (PCOS) Management Diet Cookbook, people can obtain vital insights and practical solutions for managing their symptoms and improving their overall health and well-being. Individuals with PCOS can take control of their health and thrive despite the problems they confront by eating nutritiously, exercising regularly, managing stress, and receiving support from healthcare experts and loved ones.

Understanding Blood Sugar and Insulin Regulation.

To understand the importance of blood sugar and insulin management in managing Polycystic Ovarian Syndrome (PCOS), it is critical to understand their roles in the body. Blood sugar, or glucose, is the primary energy source for cells. Insulin, a pancreatic hormone, is essential for controlling blood sugar levels. When we eat carbs, they break down into glucose, causing our blood sugar levels to rise. In reaction, the pancreas secretes insulin, which aids in the uptake of glucose into cells for energy or storage.

Insulin resistance occurs when cells become less responsive to insulin, resulting in high blood sugar levels. This condition is inextricably linked to PCOS, as many people with PCOS also have insulin resistance. The exact mechanism underlying this link is unknown, however, it is thought that hormonal imbalances in PCOS, such as high levels of androgens (male hormones), lead to insulin resistance. Furthermore, insulin resistance exacerbates PCOS symptoms by increasing androgen production, interfering with ovarian function, and encouraging weight gain.

Stabilizing blood sugar levels is critical for successful PCOS management. Fluctuations in blood sugar can develop insulin resistance, worsen hormonal imbalances, and lead to weight gain—all of which are characteristic of PCOS. Individuals with PCOS can alleviate symptoms, enhance fertility outcomes, and lower their risk of long-term consequences including type 2 diabetes and cardiovascular disease by keeping their blood sugar levels steady.

Choosing Low Glycemic Index Foods:

In PCOS management, one technique for stabilizing blood sugar levels is to prioritize low-glycemic index (GI) meals. The glycemic index assesses carbohydrate-rich foods according to their ability to spike blood sugar levels. Low GI foods slowly release glucose into the system, minimizing blood sugar spikes and crashes. Low-GI foods include non-starchy vegetables, legumes, whole grains, and fruits like berries. Individuals with PCOS can enhance insulin sensitivity and blood sugar regulation by including these foods in their diet.

Using Fiber-Rich Foods to Improve Blood Sugar Control:

Fibre helps with blood sugar regulation by decreasing glucose absorption and increasing satiety. As a result, people with PCOS must include fiber-rich foods in their diets. These foods include whole grains, vegetables, fruits, nuts, and seeds. Soluble fiber, for instance, generates a gel-like substance in the digestive tract, helping to manage blood sugar and cholesterol levels. Individuals with PCOS can improve blood sugar control and metabolic health by incorporating a range of fiber-rich foods into their diet.

Strategies to Prevent Spikes and Crashes:

One of the primary goals of PCOS therapy is to avoid blood sugar spikes and crashes. To do this, individuals might use a variety of tactics, including:

Eating Balanced Meals: Consuming balanced meals and snacks at regular intervals helps to keep blood sugar levels consistent throughout the day.

Balancing Macronutrients: Combining carbohydrates with protein, healthy fats, and fiber-rich foods will reduce glucose absorption and prevent blood sugar increases.

Limiting Refined carbs and Sugars: Refined carbs and added sugars can cause sharp changes in blood sugar levels. As a result, it is best to limit your intake of sugary beverages, pastries, white bread, and processed foods.

Monitoring Portion Sizes: Paying attention to portion sizes will help you avoid overeating, which can contribute to high glucose levels and subsequent blood sugar increases.

: Drinking plenty of water helps keep you hydrated and promotes proper metabolic function, which can lead to more stable blood sugar levels.

Incorporating these methods into a PCOS management diet cookbook can help people with PCOS gain control of their health and enhance their general well-being. A cookbook that emphasizes nutrient-dense, low-GI foods, and mindful eating techniques might be a useful resource for negotiating the dietary issues associated with PCOS.

Breakfast Boosts: Energising Morning Meals.

Breakfast is frequently seen as the most important meal of the day, and for people suffering from Polycystic Ovarian Syndrome (PCOS), it is especially significant.

Starting the day with healthy, energizing foods will help you manage your PCOS symptoms positively. A breakfast rich in whole, nutrient-dense ingredients can help stabilize blood sugar levels, promote hormone balance, and provide energy throughout the day.

CHAPTER FIVE

Quick and Easy Breakfast Options

Breakfast convenience is critical for those with PCOS. Quick and simple solutions ensure that hectic mornings do not undermine nutritional plans. These may include grab-and-go options like Greek yogurt with almonds and berries, avocado toast on whole grain bread, or a smoothie containing leafy greens, protein powder, and healthy fat. Individuals with PCOS can prioritize their health without losing time or taste by eating a simple yet nutritious breakfast.

An optimal PCOS diet emphasizes macronutrient balance, specifically protein, fiber, and healthy fats. Protein-rich foods like eggs, Greek yogurt, and lean meats assist in regulating blood sugar levels and induce fullness, lowering the likelihood of energy dips and cravings later in the day. Fiber-rich foods like fruits, vegetables, and whole grains promote digestive health and sensations of fullness, whilst healthy fats like avocados, nuts, and seeds provide long-lasting energy and support hormonal balance.

Overnight oats and smoothies are diverse breakfast options that meet the demands of people with PCOS. Overnight oats can be prepared ahead of time, providing a more convenient morning routine. Individuals can make a customizable breakfast that is both gratifying and nutritious by combining rolled oats with milk or yogurt, chia seeds, and a range of flavorful add-ins including fruits, nuts, and spices. Smoothies are another simple alternative for including leafy greens, protein, and healthy fats in your diet. With infinite flavor combinations to try, overnight oats and smoothies make it simple to start the day on a tasty and beneficial note.

Egg-Based Dishes for Sustained Energy

Eggs are a nutritious powerhouse and an especially beneficial addition to the morning menu of people with PCOS. Eggs, which are abundant in protein, vitamins, and minerals, provide long-lasting energy while also supporting muscle repair and maintenance. Incorporating egg-based foods into breakfast, such as omelets, frittatas, or hard-boiled eggs paired with whole-grain toast, provides a well-rounded meal that increases satiety and blood sugar stability. Furthermore, eggs are a versatile component that can be mixed with a variety of vegetables and herbs to produce delectable and nutritious dishes according to individual tastes and preferences.

Creative Ways to Eat Breakfast Without Refined Carbs

To assist in stabilize blood sugar levels and improving insulin resistance, people with PCOS frequently prioritize avoiding refined carbs in their diet. Fortunately, there are numerous inventive ways to consume breakfast without relying on refined carbohydrates. Cauliflower rice can be used as a low-carb substitute for regular grains in recipes like breakfast bowls and "rice" porridge. Spiralized zucchini or sweet potato noodles are a nutrient-dense alternative to breakfast pasta. Furthermore, replacing refined flour with almond flour or coconut flour in pancakes and muffins creates a grain-free option high in protein and healthy fats. Individuals with PCOS might achieve their health and well-being objectives by thinking outside the box and experimenting with new foods.

CHAPTER SIX

Lunch time Favourites: Nutrient-rich midday Meals

A well-balanced diet is essential for controlling Polycystic Ovarian Syndrome (PCOS). Lunchtime, as a crucial meal of the day, provides an opportunity to eat nutrient-dense meals that promote hormonal balance and vitality. Here are some ideas for PCOS control in the context of a lunchtime cookbook:

Colorful Salads with Lean Protein: Salads are a great way to incorporate a range of nutrient-dense veggies, which are necessary for PCOS management. Colorful vegetables such as spinach, kale, bell peppers, and carrots not only add visual appeal but also include a variety of vitamins, minerals, and antioxidants. Lean proteins like grilled chicken breast, tofu, or chickpeas can help with satiety and blood sugar regulation. Salads with healthy fats such as avocado or almonds can also help with nutrition absorption and hormone balance.

Wraps and sandwiches loaded with vegetables are versatile and convenient for midday meals. Choosing whole-grain or gluten-free wraps ensures a consistent release of energy and promotes blood sugar regulation, which is especially beneficial for those with PCOS. Fillings can include a variety of vegetables such as cucumbers, tomatoes, lettuce, and sprouts, as well as lean proteins such as turkey, salmon, or hummus for vegetarian choices. Adding tasty spreads such as pesto or avocado mash can improve taste while also providing healthy fats and nutrients.

Soups and stews make very satisfying lunches, especially during the winter months. They provide an excellent opportunity to combine a range of PCOS-friendly components, such as veggies, legumes, and lean proteins, in a single dish. Choosing broth-based soups over creamy ones helps control calorie intake while still providing adequate nutrition and hydration. Ingredients such as lentils, beans, quinoa, and lean meats or poultry can be used to increase protein content and enhance fullness. Furthermore, adding herbs and spices improves flavor while also providing anti-inflammatory and metabolic advantages.

Batch cooking is a time-saving method that can simplify meal preparation, making it simpler to stick to a PCOS-friendly diet. Individuals can prepare quick and nutritious meals throughout the week by pre-cooking big batches of fundamental components such as grains, meats, and vegetables. Preparing components like quinoa, brown rice, grilled chicken, roasted veggies, and bean salads ahead of time provides for quick customization and guarantees that healthful foods are available when time is restricted.

Incorporating Leftovers into New Dishes: Using leftovers to create new dishes is a sustainable method to reduce food waste while keeping meals interesting. Grilled chicken may be shredded and mixed into salads or wraps, while roasted vegetables can be transformed into grain bowls or frittatas. Furthermore, integrating leftovers into soups or stir-fries allows for unique flavor combinations and offers a well-balanced dinner. Individuals can support PCOS management by strategically preparing meals and utilizing leftovers.

Overall, providing nutrient-dense midday meals requires a combination of colorful whole foods, lean proteins, healthy fats, and intelligent meal planning. By adding these ideas to a PCOS management diet cookbook, people can enjoy pleasant and healthy lunches that promote hormonal balance, energy levels, and general well-being.

Dinner Delights: Healthy Evening Fare

Dinner is frequently the primary meal of the day for many people, making it an important aspect of managing Polycystic Ovarian Syndrome (PCOS) with diet. Wholesome evening fare is more than just gratifying hunger; it also provides the body with critical nutrients while keeping hormonal abnormalities linked with PCOS in line. This portion of the PCOS Management Diet Cookbook focuses on creating delicious and nutritious dinners that are tailored to the unique needs of people with PCOS.

This section has a wide variety of dishes that are not only delicious but also specifically designed to help with PCOS control. These recipes are intended to include elements that promote hormonal balance, insulin management, and overall well-being. These delicious dinners promote health and energy by emphasizing whole foods and thoughtful cooking practices.

One-pan dinners with minimum cleanup

For those with PCOS, convenience is essential, especially when it comes to meal preparation and cleanup. One-pan dinners are an excellent alternative, providing a simple cooking experience with minimum cleanup. These recipes often ask for blending

all ingredients in a single pan or pot, avoiding
the need for several dishes and utensils.

CHAPTER SEVEN

Protein alternatives include grilling, baking, and roasting.

Protein is a vital component of a healthy diet, particularly for people with PCOS. Incorporating lean protein sources into your meals can help regulate blood sugar levels, improve satiety, and support muscular health. Grilling, baking, and roasting are healthy cooking methods that enhance the natural flavors of proteins without adding too many fats or calories.

This section includes a variety of protein alternatives produced with these cooking techniques. From luscious grilled chicken breasts to soft baked fish fillets, these recipes provide delectable ways to integrate protein into your evening routine. By selecting lean cuts of meat, chicken, or fish and mixing them with tasty herbs and spices, you can create satisfying meals that help you control PCOS.

Vegetable-focused dinners for Variety

Vegetables are crucial components of any balanced diet, especially for people with PCOS. Vegetables are high in vitamins, minerals, and fiber, which aid digestion and supply critical nutrients for overall health. Creating vegetable-centric dinners is an excellent method to increase your intake of these healthy foods while also adding variety and flavor to your meals.

This section features a variety of recipes that highlight the natural flavors and textures of vegetables. From colorful salads to substantial vegetable stir-fries, these recipes highlight the variety of plant-based ingredients. By combining a variety of veggies into your dinners, you can create meals that are both delicious and nutritious for your health.

Comforting casseroles and skillet dinners.

Comfort food does not have to be bad, especially if you are treating PCOS. Casseroles and skillet meals are traditional comfort foods that may simply be modified to fit into a healthy diet. You may enjoy these comfortable meals without jeopardizing your health goals by using healthful products and limiting your portion sizes.

Mindful eating habits for supper

Mindful eating is a key part of controlling PCOS and improving overall health. By paying attention to your body's hunger and fullness cues, you may improve your relationship with food and make more informed decisions about what and how much you eat. Dinnertime provides an excellent opportunity to practice mindful eating and develop a stronger relationship with your food.

In this section, you will learn about numerous mindful eating strategies that can help you enjoy your supper more while also supporting your PCOS management goals.

Taking the time to savor each bite and paying attention to how different foods make you feel are two habits that can help you create a stronger feeling of awareness and contentment during mealtimes. By introducing mindfulness into your dinner practice, you can improve your entire eating experience and assist your PCOS-related health journey.

Snack Attack: Smart Options for Between Meals

Snacking can be an important part of controlling Polycystic Ovarian Syndrome (PCOS) since it helps control blood sugar levels and prevent energy dumps. The idea is to make informed decisions that promote hormonal balance and general wellness. Here's an in-depth look at numerous snacking strategies for PCOS management:

Balanced Snack Ideas to Reduce Cravings: Balance is key when snacking with PCOS. To keep you full and your blood sugar levels stable, choose snacks that contain protein, healthy fats, and fiber. Opt for munchies like:

Greek yogurt with berries: Greek yogurt has protein, while berries contain fiber and antioxidants.

Apple slices with almond butter: Apples give fiber, while almond butter contains healthy fats and protein.

Hummus with carrot sticks: Hummus contains protein and healthy fats, while carrot sticks provide fiber and crunch.

Cottage cheese is high in protein, and pineapple contains natural sweetness and vitamin C.

Avocado on whole grain toast: Avocado has healthy fats, and whole grain toast contains fiber and complex carbohydrates.

Portion control strategies for snacking: Portion control is essential for managing PCOS because overeating can contribute to weight gain and worsen symptoms. Here are some tips to help you practice portion management while snacking:

Portion out foods ahead of time using tiny dishes or containers.

Avoid eating directly from large bags or containers since portion sizes can be difficult to keep track of.

Instead of eating until you're full, listen to your hunger cues and quit when you're content.

To avoid overconsumption, measure out quantities of snacks, especially those high in calories like nuts or dried fruit.

Be cautious of the serving sizes mentioned on food packages and stick to the recommended portions.

CHAPTER EIGHT

Including enough vegetables in your snacks is critical for obtaining crucial nutrients and fiber. Pairing vegetables with nutritious dips and spreads can make them more appealing. Here are a few ideas:

Guacamole with cucumber slices: Guacamole is created with avocado, which contains healthful fats, while cucumber slices provide crispness and hydration.

Tzatziki with bell pepper strips: Tzatziki is a protein-rich yogurt dip, while bell pepper strips contain vitamin C and fiber.

Salsa with jicama sticks: Salsa is low in calories and high in flavor, while jicama sticks add a refreshing crunch.

Peanut butter with celery sticks: Peanut butter contains protein and healthy fats, whereas celery sticks are hydrating and low in calories.

Bean dip with cherry tomatoes: Bean dip is high in protein and fiber, while cherry tomatoes provide sweetness and antioxidants.

Homemade Trail Mix with Energy Bites: Trail mix and energy bites are practical snacks that may be tailored to your taste preferences and nutritional requirements. Making them at home gives you control over the ingredients and eliminates extra sweets and preservatives. Here are a few ideas:

Trail mix with nuts, seeds, and dried fruit: Mix almonds, walnuts, pumpkin seeds, and dried cranberries for a well-balanced snack high in protein, healthy fat, and antioxidants.

Energy bites with oats, nut butter, and honey: Combine rolled oats, almond butter, honey, and dark chocolate chips to make bite-sized snacks that provide long-lasting energy while satisfying sweet cravings.

Coconut bliss balls: Combine dates, shredded coconut, almond flour, and vanilla extract to form healthful and tasty energy balls that are ideal foSr on-the-go snacks.

Almond joy trail mix: Combine almonds, coconut flakes, dark chocolate chips, and dried cherries to make a delicious and delightful snack inspired by the traditional sweet bar.

Protcin-packed energy balls: Combine protein powder, almond butter, oats, and honey to make high-protein energy balls that promote muscle recovery and keep you satisfied in between meals.

Processed snacks and sugary desserts can disrupt blood sugar levels and exacerbate PCOS symptoms. It's critical to minimize these items and choose healthy alternatives wherever possible. Here are some ways to avoid processed snacks and sugary treats:

Read food labels carefully and avoid items with added sugars, artificial sweeteners, and preservatives.

Choose entire foods with little processing, such as fruits, vegetables, nuts, seeds, and whole grains.

Make homemade snacks and treats from natural foods such as fruits, nuts, seeds, and whole grains.

Keep harmful snacks out of sight and stock your kitchen with nutritional options to make healthy eating simpler.

Practice mindful eating by paying attention to how different foods make you feel, then choose foods that nourish your body and promote your overall well-being.

By implementing balanced snack ideas, exercising portion control, enjoying nutritious dips and spreads with vegetables, making homemade trail mix and energy bites, and avoiding processed snacks and sugary sweets, you may help manage PCOS and enhance overall health and well-being. Remember to pay attention to your body's hunger and fullness cues and make decisions that reflect your unique dietary needs and preferences.

Sweet Treats: Guiltless Desserts & Sweets

Diet is important for controlling Polycystic Ovarian Syndrome (PCOS). A successful PCOS treatment diet cookbook should contain a section on sweet treats, providing choices that are not only delicious but also beneficial to hormonal balance and general wellness. Let's look into the numerous themes in this part.

Fruit-based sweets provide natural sweetness while also providing a variety of vitamins, minerals, and fiber. Individuals with PCOS can fulfill cravings by choosing fruit-based treats that do not cause blood sugar rises. Fruit salads, fruit parfaits, grilled fruits drizzled with honey, and baked apples with cinnamon are all examples of recipes in this category. These sweets satisfy your sweet tooth while also increasing your daily fruit intake and maintaining stable blood sugar levels.

Low-carb baking alternatives: Traditional baked goods are frequently loaded with refined carbohydrates, which can increase insulin resistance in PCOS patients. Low-carb baking substitutes refined flour and sugars with nutrient-dense foods that have a lesser effect on blood sugar levels. Recipes may call for almond flour, coconut flour, or flaxseed meal in place of wheat flour, as well as natural sweeteners such as stevia or monk fruit in place of refined sugar. From muffins and cookies to cakes and bread, these options allow people with PCOS to enjoy baked goods without jeopardizing their dietary goals.

does not have to imply forsaking nutrition. This section contains recipes that find a balance between indulgence and health by using ingredients high in critical nutrients. For example, chocolate avocado mousse has a creamy, delicious texture while also containing heart-healthy fats and antioxidants. Nut butter energy balls are a deliciously sweet snack high in protein and fiber. Individuals with PCOS can enjoy snacks that feed their health while also gratifying their sweet desires by carefully selecting components.

Portion management and conscious indulgence: While savoring sweet foods is an important part of any diet, portion control is essential, especially for people with PCOS who are sensitive to blood sugar changes. This section emphasizes the significance of mindful eating and provides solutions for quantity control.

Recipes may include advice on serving amounts, how to enjoy each bite thoughtfully, and how to recognize hunger and fullness cues. Individuals with PCOS can enjoy their favorite sweets without jeopardizing their nutritional goals by practicing portion management and mindful pleasure.

Celebrating special occasions with healthier desserts: While special occasions sometimes call for celebratory desserts, people with

PCOS do not have to sacrifice their health goals.

This section of the cookbook contains recipes for healthier adaptations of classic delicacies to be enjoyed on special occasions. Whether it's a birthday cake, Christmas cookies, or festive pies, these recipes emphasize nutrient-dense foods and careful preparation without losing flavor or enjoyment. The cookbook encourages people with PCOS to celebrate without guilt by providing healthier alternatives for special occasions while staying on track with their nutritional requirements.

In summary, the "Sweet Treats" section of a PCOS management diet cookbook provides a choice of dessert alternatives tailored to the dietary needs and preferences of people with PCOS. From fruit-based delights to indulgent yet healthy treats, these recipes promote stable blood sugar levels, hormonal balance, and general well-being, allowing people with PCOS to indulge guilt-free while also supporting their health goals.

Quinoa meal Bowl with Berries and Almonds: This protein-packed meal is high in fiber and antioxidants, which help manage blood sugar levels.

Salmon and Avocado Salad: This tasty salad contains omega-3 fatty acids from salmon and healthy fats from avocado, which promote hormonal balance.

Vegetable Stir-Fry with Tofu is a colorful and nutritious dish full of fiber-rich veggies and plant-based protein from tofu.

Turkey & Vegetable Soup: This substantial soup is packed with lean protein from turkey and a variety of veggies, giving critical nutrients and aiding with weight management.

A filling and nutritious dessert or snack full of fiber, healthy fats, and antioxidants.

Mediterranean Chickpea Salad: A refreshing salad made with chickpeas, vegetables, olives, and feta cheese, which is high in fiber and plant-based protein.

Sweet Potato and Black Bean Tacos: Flavorful tacos made with sweet potatoes, black beans, and avocado, with a good balance of carbohydrates, protein, and healthy fats.

Spinach and Mushroom Stuffed Chicken Breast: This tasty and protein-rich recipe consists of lean chicken breast stuffed with spinach and mushrooms, which provides critical nutrients while also supporting hormone balance.

Greek Yoghurt Parfait with Granola and Honey: A delightful and calcium-rich breakfast or snack made with Greek yogurt, granola, and honey, which promotes bone health and provides probiotics for the gut.

Lentil & Vegetable Curry: A tasty curry dish made with lentils, veggies, and aromatic spices that provides a good dose of plant-based protein and fiber.

Let's create a 30-day meal plan for PCOS sufferers utilizing these recipes:

Day 1:

Breakfast: Quinoa bowl with berries and almonds.

Snack: Greek yogurt parfait with granola and honey.

Lunch: Vegetable Stir-Fry with Tofu.

Snack: Mixed nuts.

Dinner: Salmon and avocado salad.

Day 2:

Breakfast: Chia seed pudding with mixed berries.

Snack: Carrot Sticks and Hummus.

Lunch: Mediterranean Chickpea Salad.

Snack: Apple slices and almond butter.

Dinner is lentil and vegetable curry with brown rice.

Continue this pattern for 30 days, combining the meals to provide variety and balanced nutrition while helping with PCOS management. To get the best health outcomes, adjust portion sizes and snacks based on individual needs and tastes, and encourage regular physical exercise in addition to food adjustments.

Finally, "Polycystic Ovarian Syndrome (PCOS) Management Diet Cookbook" provides thorough guidance for people navigating the dietary complications of PCOS. Recognizing the importance of nutrition in controlling PCOS symptoms, this cookbook provides a multitude of nutrient-dense recipes designed to promote hormonal balance, weight management, and general well-being.

Throughout this cookbook, the emphasis is not just on wonderful flavors, but also on the nutritional value of each dish. Every cuisine, from protein-packed breakfast bowls to vivid salads brimming with antioxidants, is deliberately designed to deliver critical nutrients while adhering to the dietary recommendations for PCOS control.

Furthermore, the 30-day meal plan presented in this cookbook provides structure and assistance for anyone looking to make effective nutritional adjustments. Readers can experience the benefits of a balanced diet firsthand by including a varied assortment of dishes over 30 days, thereby supporting their journey to improved health and symptom management.

Beyond the meals, this cookbook promotes a holistic approach to PCOS care. Recognizing the interdependence of nutrition, lifestyle, and hormonal balance, readers are advised to supplement their dietary adjustments with regular physical activity, stress management skills, and appropriate sleep.

Furthermore, the cookbook's educational tools and practical suggestions enable readers to make informed health decisions. From understanding the role of carbohydrates in insulin resistance to analyzing food labels for hidden sugars, readers will receive essential knowledge to help them continue their

nutritional journey beyond the pages of this
cookbook.

In essence, "Polycystic Ovarian Syndrome
(PCOS) Management Diet Cookbook" is a
reliable companion for those navigating the
dietary obstacles of PCOS. With a variety of
delicious recipes, structured meal plans, and
practical advice, this cookbook provides
readers with the tools they need to take
control of their health and thrive on their
path to PCOS treatment.

THE END

www.ingramcontent.com/pod-product-compliance
Lightning Source LLC
Chambersburg PA
CBHW061254250726
48653CB00002B/663